FIBROMYALGIA DIET COOKBOOK FOR VEGETARIANS

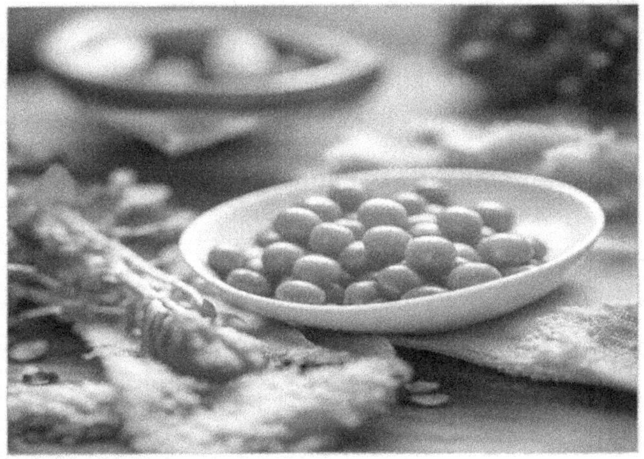

The complete guide to reduce pain and inflammation with delicious and nutrition recipes.

KATHLEEN G MARION

TABLE OF CONTENT

INTRODUCTION

ay's Symphony of Relief: A Vegetarian's Dance with Fibromyalgia

Jay, a man woven from music, used to conduct the orchestra of his life with vibrant energy. But a discordant note crept in - fibromyalgia. Aching muscles, chronic fatigue, and brain fog transformed his once lively melody into a melancholic dirge. He embarked on a desperate search for harmony, trying various diets, each a failed experiment leaving him frustrated and deflated.

One rainy afternoon, amidst sheet music and despair, Jay stumbled upon a beacon of hope - your Fibromyalgia Diet Cookbook for Vegetarians. Skepticism lingered, but the promise of plant-based solutions resonated with his compassionate nature. Hesitantly, he opened the book, and its pages unfolded like a symphony, each recipe a movement promising relief.

He started with a simple breakfast of almond butter and chia seed pudding, the creamy sweetness a gentle awakening for his body. Lunch became a vibrant concerto of roasted vegetables and quinoa, the colors as cheerful as a Beethoven sonata. Dinners transformed into grand finales, tofu curries and lentil stews bursting with flavor, nourishing his body and soul.

The changes were subtle at first, like a hesitant oboe joining the melody. The achy symphony began to soften, replaced by a gentle hum of well-being. He had more energy to climb the stairs, the brain fog thinned, and a smile, long absent, reappeared on his face. He wasn't just eating food; he was conducting a symphony of healing within his own body.

The book wasn't just a collection of recipes; it was a guide, a conductor leading him through the complex score of his condition. He learned about anti-inflammatory ingredients, the importance of gut health, and the power of mindful eating. Each delicious bite became a note of gratitude, a testament to his newfound control.

One sunny morning, Jay sat down at his piano, fingers tentatively caressing the keys. The music flowed, no longer a struggle but a joyous expression. He had found his harmony, not just in the music, but in his body and mind. He wasn't cured, but he was empowered, the conductor of his own well-being, playing a vibrant melody of life.

Jay's story is a testament to the transformative power of food and knowledge. If you're struggling with the discordant notes of fibromyalgia, consider picking up your own copy of this life-changing cookbook. It might just be the missing instrument in your own symphony of healing. Remember, you are the conductor of your health, and the music awaits your touch.

CHAPTER 1

Fibromyalgia, a chronic condition characterized by widespread pain, fatigue, and other symptoms, can feel like a discordant note in the symphony of life. But for vegetarians, navigating the often meat-centric recommendations for managing fibromyalgia can be even more challenging. This guide, inspired by your Fibromyalgia Diet Cookbook for Vegetarians, aims to empower you with knowledge and delicious solutions, transforming food into your ally in managing fibromyalgia and reclaiming your well-being.

Understanding the Many Faces of Fibromyalgia:

Fibromyalgia isn't a one-size-fits-all condition. It manifests in various forms, each with its own nuances:

- **generalized pain**: Aching, burning, or throbbing pain throughout the body, often worse in the morning or after periods of inactivity.

- **Fatigue:** A persistent feeling of exhaustion, even after sleeping adequately.

- **Sleep disturbances**: Difficulty falling asleep, staying asleep, or experiencing unrefreshing sleep.

- **Cognitive difficulties**: Problems with memory, concentration, and focus, often referred to as "fibro fog."

- **Mood changes**: Increased anxiety, depression, or emotional sensitivity.

While the exact cause of fibromyalgia remains a mystery, research suggests a complex interplay of factors:

- **Genetics**: Certain genes might make individuals more susceptible.

- **Neurotransmitters**: Imbalances in brain chemicals like serotonin and dopamine might contribute to pain and mood changes.

- **Central nervous system**: Abnormal pain processing in the brain and spinal cord could be involved.

- **Stress and trauma**: Physical or emotional stress can trigger or worsen symptoms.

Recognizing the Discordant Notes: Symptoms to Watch Out For:

While pain is the most commonly recognized symptom, fibromyalgia presents a wider range:

- **Widespread pain**: Pain lasting at least three months in various areas of the body, including the back, neck, shoulders, hips, and legs.

- **Tenderness:** Increased sensitivity to touch in specific points on your body.

- **Fatigue**: Feeling exhausted and drained even after a good night's sleep.

- **Sleep disturbances**: Difficulty falling asleep, staying asleep, or experiencing unrefreshing sleep.

- **Morning stiffness**: Feeling stiff and achy upon waking up, which improves with movement?

- **Cognitive difficulties**: Memory problems, difficulty concentrating, and brain fog.

- **Headaches**: Migraines or tension headaches.

- **Mood changes**: Anxiety, depression, or irritability.

- **Numbness or tingling**: Tingling or numb sensations in hands or feet.

- **Irritable bowel syndrome (IBS)**: Digestive issues like bloating, constipation, or diarrhea.

Silencing the Discordance: Preventive Measures for a More Harmonious Life:

While there's no cure for fibromyalgia, proactive steps can significantly manage symptoms and improve your quality of life:

- **Manage stress**: Practice relaxation techniques like yoga, meditation, or deep breathing to reduce stress, a known trigger for flares.

- **Get enough sleep**: Aim for 7-8 hours of quality sleep each night to promote both physical and mental well-being.

- **Stay active**: Regular exercise, even low-impact activities like walking or swimming, can improve pain, fatigue, and sleep.

- **Maintain a healthy weight**: Excess weight can worsen fibromyalgia symptoms, so focus on a balanced diet and regular exercise.

- **Build a strong support system**: Surround yourself with supportive friends, family, and healthcare professionals who can provide emotional and practical help.

The Vegetarian's Culinary Symphony: Food as Your Ally:

Your Fibromyalgia Diet Cookbook for Vegetarians goes beyond bland restrictions. It offers a delicious and effective approach to managing fibromyalgia through targeted vegetarian nutrition:

- **Anti-inflammatory Diet**: This approach prioritizes fruits, vegetables, whole grains, lean protein sources like beans and lentils, and healthy fats like nuts and seeds, while minimizing inflammatory foods like processed meats, sugary drinks, and refined carbohydrates.

- **Recipes Tailored to Your Needs**: Discover a symphony of dishes catering to diverse vegetarian preferences, offering delicious alternatives to potential triggers.

- **Meal Plans**: Take the guesswork out of healthy eating with weekly plans designed to support your fibromyalgia management journey.

- **Expert Guidance**: Gain insights from medical professionals and chefs, empowering you to navigate dietary choices with confidence.

CHAPTER 2

Living **with fibromyalgia** can feel like conducting an orchestra with off-key instruments – pain, fatigue, and other symptoms disrupt the melody of your life. Yet, just like tuning the instruments, dietary changes can transform the discord into a symphony of well-being. Your Fibromyalgia Diet Cookbook for Vegetarians empowers you to achieve this transformation by focusing on the "right notes" - foods that nourish and minimize the "wrong notes" that exacerbate symptoms.

Embracing the Anti-inflammatory Chorus:

Imagine a vibrant plate bursting with colors – your anti-inflammatory haven. These ingredients become your allies, reducing inflammation, a potential contributor to fibromyalgia symptoms:

- **Fruits and Vegetables**: Nature's powerhouses, rich in antioxidants and vitamins, like berries, leafy greens, peppers, and citrus fruits.

- **Whole Grains**: Choose brown rice, quinoa, oats, and whole-wheat bread for sustained energy and fiber.

- **Lean Protein**: Opt for plant-based options like beans, lentils, tofu, tempeh, nuts, and seeds for essential nutrients without inflammatory effects.

- **Healthy Fats**: Embrace avocados, nuts, seeds, and olive oil as sources of good fats crucial for brain health and inflammation reduction.

- **Spices and Herbs**: Explore the anti-inflammatory properties of turmeric, ginger, garlic, and rosemary to add flavor and boost your health.

Identifying the Discordant Notes:

While every individual's trigger landscape is unique, certain ingredients are known to disrupt the harmony for some:

- **Processed Meats**: Hot dogs, sausages, and deli meats often contain nitrates and nitrites, potential triggers for some individuals.

- **Refined Carbohydrates**: White bread, sugary cereals, and pastries cause blood sugar spikes linked to fatigue and other symptoms.

- **Dairy Products**: While some tolerate dairy well, others find that it worsens pain and inflammation. Consider exploring plant-based alternatives like almond or oat milk.

- **Gluten**: If you have gluten sensitivity, it's crucial to avoid wheat, barley, and rye to prevent digestive issues and inflammation.

- **Certain Vegetables**: Nightshade vegetables like tomatoes, potatoes, peppers, and eggplant can trigger inflammation for some individuals. Monitor your response and adjust accordingly.

Beyond "Don't Eat": Creative Substitutions:

Your Fibromyalgia Diet Cookbook for Vegetarians doesn't just tell you what to avoid; it empowers you with a delicious world of alternatives:

- Craving pizza? Swap processed dough for a whole-wheat cauliflower crust, top it with grilled tempeh or vegetables.

- Need a sweet treat? Indulge in a smoothie made with berries, spinach, and almond milk for a satisfying and nutritious burst.

- Yearning for comfort food? Whip up a lentil soup packed with protein and fiber, seasoned with fragrant herbs.

Beyond Food: A Holistic Approach to Harmony:

While diet plays a crucial role, remember that managing fibromyalgia involves a multi-faceted approach:

- **Stress Management**: Techniques like yoga, meditation, and deep breathing can significantly reduce stress, a known trigger for flares.

- **Regular Exercise**: Aim for low-impact activities like walking, swimming, or gentle yoga to improve pain, fatigue, and sleep.

- **Quality Sleep**: Prioritize 7-8 hours of uninterrupted sleep each night to promote both physical and mental well-being.

- **Supportive Network**: Surround yourself with people who understand and support your journey, offering emotional and practical help.

CHAPTER 3

Core Benefits of Following a Fibromyalgia Diet Cookbook for Vegetarians:

Reduced Pain and Inflammation:

- **Anti-inflammatory focus**: Prioritizing fruits, vegetables, whole grains, and plant-based protein sources reduces inflammation, potentially contributing to less pain and stiffness.

- **Identification and avoidance of triggers**: Eliminating individual trigger foods can significantly decrease pain flares and improve overall well-being.

- **Increased nutrient intake**: A balanced diet ensures essential vitamins and minerals crucial for managing pain and supporting your immune system.

Improved Energy and Sleep:

- **Balanced blood sugar**: Minimizing refined carbohydrates prevents blood sugar spikes and crashes, leading to more sustained energy throughout the day.

- **Gut health promotion**: The focus on fiber-rich foods supports a healthy gut microbiome, impacting energy levels and sleep quality.

- **Reduced fatigue**: Anti-inflammatory dietary choices can combat fatigue, a common symptom of fibromyalgia.

Enhanced Mood and Cognitive Function:

- **Nutrient support**: Essential vitamins and minerals like B vitamins and omega-3 fatty acids are crucial for brain health and mood regulation.

- **Reduced inflammation**: Chronic inflammation can negatively impact mood and cognitive function. Addressing it through diet can offer significant benefits.

- **Improved sleep**: Quality sleep is vital for cognitive function and emotional well-being. The dietary approach promotes better sleep patterns.

Lifestyle and Management Benefits:

- **Empowerment and control**: Taking charge of your diet fosters a sense of control over your health and empowers you to manage your fibromyalgia.

- **Weight management**: Maintaining a healthy weight can lessen the burden on your joints and potentially reduce pain.

- **Sustainability and variety**: The vegetarian approach offers countless delicious and fulfilling meal options, promoting long-term adherence.

- **Improved overall health**: Embracing a healthy lifestyle through dietary changes often leads to positive impacts on heart health, blood pressure, and overall well-being.

Personalized Approach and Support:

- **Tailored guidance**: Consulting a dietitian can personalize the plan based on your specific needs, preferences, and trigger foods.

- **Community and support**: Online communities and support groups can offer encouragement, share experiences, and provide valuable insights.

- **Holistic approach**: Remember, diet is just one piece of the puzzle. Combining it with stress management, sleep hygiene, and regular exercise maximizes benefits.

CHAPTER 4

While I can't give specific medical advice, I can offer some general guidance on following a fibromyalgia diet cookbook for vegetarians:

Before you start:

- **Consult your doctor**: Discuss any dietary changes with your doctor first, especially if you have other health conditions or take medications.

- **Choose a reputable cookbook**: Look for resources with evidence-based information and recipes created by registered dietitians or other qualified healthcare professionals familiar with fibromyalgia and vegetarian diets.

- **Consider your individual needs**: Be mindful of any food sensitivities or allergies you may have. Pay attention to how different foods affect your symptoms and adjust your diet accordingly.

Following the cookbook:

- **Start gradually**: Don't make drastic changes all at once. Introduce new foods gradually to see how your body reacts.

- **Focus on anti-inflammatory foods**: Prioritize fruits, vegetables, whole grains, legumes, nuts, and seeds, known for their anti-inflammatory properties.

- **Limit inflammatory foods**: Reduce or avoid processed foods, refined carbohydrates, sugary drinks, red meat, saturated and Trans fats, as these can worsen inflammation.

- **Read labels carefully**: Pay attention to added sugars, sodium, and unhealthy fats in packaged foods.

- **Stay hydrated**: Drink plenty of water throughout the day to stay hydrated and support overall health.

- **Cook at home when possible**: This allows you to control ingredients and portion sizes.

- **Plan and prep meals**: Planning and prepping meals in advance can make it easier to stick to your diet, especially during flares.

- **be patient and consistent**: It takes time to see results from any dietary changes. Stick with it and be patient with yourself.

CHAPTER 5

Fruits and Vegetables:

1.   **Leafy greens**: Kale, spinach, Swiss chard, collard greens (rich in antioxidants and anti-inflammatory nutrients)

2.   **Berries**: Blueberries, strawberries, raspberries (high in antioxidants and fiber)

3.   **Bell peppers**: Red, yellow, orange (rich in vitamin C and antioxidants)

4.   **Fatty fish**: Salmon, tuna (for vegetarians, consider flaxseeds or chia seeds for omega-3s)

5.   **Cruciferous vegetables**: Broccoli, cauliflower, Brussels sprouts (rich in antioxidants and sulforaphane)

6.   **Citrus fruits**: Oranges, grapefruits, lemons (high in vitamin C and fiber)

7.   **Nuts and seeds**: Almonds, walnuts, chia seeds, flaxseeds (healthy fats, protein, and fiber)

8.   **Legumes**: Lentils, black beans, chickpeas (plant-based protein and fiber)

9.   **Avocados**: (healthy fats, fiber, and vitamins)

10.   **Ginger and turmeric**: (anti-inflammatory properties)

Pantry Staples:

11.   **Whole grains**: Brown rice, quinoa, oats, barley (fiber, complex carbohydrates)

12.   **Olive oil**: Extra virgin (healthy fats and antioxidants)

13.   **Spices**: Turmeric, ginger, garlic, black pepper (anti-inflammatory properties and flavor)

14.   **Vinegar:** Apple cider vinegar, balsamic vinegar (adds flavor and aids digestion)

15.   **Unsweetened plant-based milk**: Almond milk, soy milk, oat milk (calcium and vitamin D)

16.   **Eggs:** (protein and choline)

17.   **Nutritional yeast**: (vitamin B12 and protein)

18.   **Dried fruits**: Unsweetened cranberries, raisins (fiber and antioxidants)

19.   **Seeds**: Pumpkin seeds, sunflower seeds (healthy fats and protein)

20.   **Herbal teas**: Chamomile, ginger, peppermint (calming and digestive properties).

CHAPTER 6

While a well-planned vegetarian diet can offer numerous benefits for managing fibromyalgia symptoms, there are potential complications if the right approach isn't adopted. Here are some key points to consider:

Nutrient Deficiencies:

- **Protein**: Plant-based protein sources can be excellent, but careful planning is crucial to ensure adequate protein intake for muscle health and energy levels.

- **Iron**: Vegetarian diets can be lower in iron, which is important for fatigue management and overall well-being. Including iron-rich plant sources like lentils, leafy greens, and fortified foods is essential.

- **Omega-3 fatty acids**: These facts are crucial for managing inflammation. While vegetarians can get them from flaxseeds, chia seeds, and walnuts, some may benefit from supplementation.

- **Vitamin B12**: This vitamin is only readily available in animal sources. Vegetarians need to ensure adequate intake through fortified foods, nutritional yeast, or supplements.

Increased Inflammation:

- **FODMAPs**: Some people with fibromyalgia are sensitive to FODMAPs, fermentable carbohydrates found in many fruits, vegetables, and grains. Ignoring this sensitivity could worsen symptoms like bloating and pain.

- **Gluten**: While not specific to fibromyalgia, some individuals might have gluten sensitivity, which can contribute to pain and fatigue. Choosing gluten-free options if necessary is crucial.

Other Complications:

- Disordered eating: Restrictive diets or focusing solely on weight loss can be detrimental to physical and mental health. Prioritize a balanced and enjoyable approach.

- **Social challenges**: Navigating social situations with dietary restrictions can be challenging. Finding supportive communities and planning ahead can help.

- **Individual needs**: Every individual with fibromyalgia is different, and responses to dietary changes can vary. Working with a registered dietitian can help tailor a plan for optimal results.

CHAPTER 7

Tailoring Vegetarian Meal Plans for Fibromyalgia: A Cookbook Author's Guide

As a cookbook author crafting vegetarian meals for individuals with fibromyalgia, understanding the distinct benefits and potential pitfalls of meal planning is crucial. This approach can empower readers to actively manage their symptoms through dietary choices while ensuring enjoyment and variety.

Benefits of Meal Planning for Fibromyalgia:

- **Targeted Anti-inflammatory Nutrition**: Prioritizing ingredients like leafy greens, berries, fatty fish (or plant-based Omega-3 sources), and spices like turmeric can significantly dampen inflammation, a key culprit in fibromyalgia pain and fatigue.

- **Enhanced Energy Regulation**: Balanced meals with protein, complex carbohydrates, and healthy fats provide sustained energy, minimizing the energy crashes commonly experienced with fibromyalgia.

- **Improved Sleep Quality**: Consistent meal timings and balanced nutrition contribute to deeper sleep, essential for managing pain and fatigue.

- **Mood Stabilization**: Regulated blood sugar levels achieved through meal planning help address mood swings and emotional volatility associated with fibromyalgia.

- **Gut Health Support**: Including fermented vegetables, fiber-rich options, and prebiotics can nurture gut health, further supporting overall well-being.

- **Reduced Stress and Burden**: Meal planning eliminates the daily stress of "what to eat," freeing up mental energy and promoting overall well-being.

Key Strategies for Professional Cookbook Development:

- **Collaborate with Healthcare Professionals**: Partner with registered dietitians and healthcare professionals to ensure evidence-based meal plans aligned with current dietary interventions for fibromyalgia.

- Personalization: Highlight the importance of individualization, acknowledging that trigger foods and dietary needs vary. Encourage readers to identify and manage personal triggers.

- **Variety and Balance**: Showcase diverse vegetarian protein sources, colorful fruits and vegetables, and whole grains to ensure nutrient adequacy and prevent culinary monotony.

- **Portion Control Guidance**: Offer portion control recommendations to promote healthy weight management and blood sugar control.

- **Simple Preparations**: Feature recipes with minimal ingredients and cooking steps, considering potential fatigue management challenges.

- **Batch Cooking Optimization**: Include tips for preparing larger portions and freezing options to save time and ensure healthy options are readily available.

- **Community and Support**: Encourage readers to share meal planning and preparation with loved ones for additional support and social interaction.

Additional Tips for Professionalism:

- **Cite Credible Sources**: Reference evidence-based research and professional guidance from dietitians and healthcare professionals throughout your cookbook.

- **Clarity and Accessibility**: Use clear, concise language and visually appealing recipe layouts for reader-friendliness.

- **Be Mindful of Scope**: Focus on providing practical and manageable meal plans while acknowledging the need for individualization and consultation with healthcare professionals for complex cases.

CHAPTER 8

Disclaimer: This is a sample meal plan and should not be considered a substitute for professional medical advice. Always consult with your doctor or a registered dietitian before making significant changes to your diet.

Remember:

- Individual needs and sensitivities vary. Pay attention to your body and adjust the plan accordingly.

- Feel free to substitute ingredients based on your preferences and dietary restrictions.

- Batch cook larger portions and freeze them for convenience.

- Include plenty of water and herbal teas throughout the day.

Day 1:

- Breakfast: Oatmeal with berries, chia seeds, and almond milk

- Lunch: Lentil soup with whole-wheat bread and a side salad

- Dinner: Tofu scramble with vegetables and brown rice

Day 2:

- Breakfast: Smoothie with spinach, banana, almond milk, and protein powder

- Lunch: Black bean burger on a whole-wheat bun with sweet potato fries

- Dinner: Vegetarian chili with quinoa and cornbread

Day 3:

- Breakfast: Eggs with avocado toast and a side of fruit

- Lunch: Chickpea salad sandwich on whole-wheat bread with cucumber and tomato

- Dinner: Vegetable stir-fry with brown rice and tofu

Day 4:

- Breakfast: Greek yogurt with fruit, granola, and honey

- Lunch: Leftover veggie chili with a side salad

- Dinner: Lentil pasta with tomato sauce and roasted vegetables

Day 5:

- Breakfast: Pancakes made with whole-wheat flour and topped with fruit and maple syrup

- Lunch: Veggie wrap with hummus, avocado, and whole-wheat tortilla

- Dinner: Vegetarian pizza with whole-wheat crust and vegetable toppings

Day 6:

- Breakfast: Chia pudding with almond milk, fruit, and nuts

- Lunch: Black bean and corn salad with avocado and quinoa

- Dinner: Tofu curry with brown rice and vegetables

Day 7:

- Breakfast: Scrambled eggs with spinach and whole-wheat toast

- Lunch: Leftover vegetarian pizza with a side salad

- Dinner: Lentil Shepherd's Pie with mashed potatoes

Day 8:

- Breakfast: Smoothie with kale, banana, almond milk, and protein powder

- Lunch: Chickpea salad sandwich on whole-wheat bread with avocado

- Dinner: Vegetarian lasagna with whole-wheat noodles and ricotta cheese

Day 9:

- Breakfast: Oatmeal with nuts, seeds, and fruit

- Lunch: Black bean soup with whole-wheat bread and a side salad

- Dinner: Tofu stir-fry with brown rice and vegetables

Day 10:

- Breakfast: Eggs with whole-wheat toast and avocado

- Lunch: Veggie wrap with hummus, cucumber, and whole-wheat tortilla

- Dinner: Vegetarian chili with quinoa and cornbread

Day 11:

- Breakfast: Greek yogurt with fruit, granola, and honey

- Lunch: Leftover vegetarian lasagna with a side salad

- Dinner: Lentil pasta with marinara sauce and grilled vegetables

Day 12:

- Breakfast: Smoothie with spinach, banana, almond milk, and protein powder

- Lunch: Black bean burger on a whole-wheat bun with sweet potato fries

- Dinner: Vegetarian tacos with corn tortillas, black beans, salsa, and avocado

Day 13:

- Breakfast: Chia pudding with almond milk, fruit, and nuts

- Lunch: Chickpea salad sandwich on whole-wheat bread with tomato and sprouts

- Dinner: Tofu curry with brown rice and vegetables

Day 14:

- Breakfast: Scrambled eggs with vegetables and whole-wheat toast

- Lunch: Leftover vegetarian tacos with a side salad

- Dinner: Lentil soup with whole-wheat bread and a side salad

CONCLUSION

Embracing Your Journey: A Final Note on Thriving with Vegetarian Fibromyalgia Cuisine

As you reach the culmination of this culinary adventure, remember, this is not just a cookbook – it's a stepping stone to a vibrant and empowered life. You've explored delicious vegetarian meals bursting with anti-inflammatory goodness, learned valuable meal planning strategies, and gained insights into tailoring this approach to your unique needs. But remember, the true magic lies in putting it all into practice.

Think of this cookbook as your compass, guiding you towards a future filled with reduced pain, enhanced energy, and improved sleep. Each recipe is a chance to nourish your body and soul, a celebration of the incredible potential within plant-based ingredients. Embrace the journey, savor the flavors, and witness the positive transformations that unfold, bite by delicious bite.

Remember, adopting a new dietary approach can be daunting, but don't let initial challenges deter you. Start small, incorporate one or two recipes into your weekly routine, and gradually expand your repertoire. Every step forward, no matter how seemingly insignificant, is a victory. Celebrate your progress, big or small, and remember, even minor adjustments can yield significant results in managing your fibromyalgia.

As you embark on this culinary adventure, remember these key takeaways:

- **Listen to your body**: It's your unique guide. Pay attention to how specific ingredients or meals affect you, and adjust accordingly.

- **Embrace variety**: Explore a kaleidoscope of flavors and textures with diverse vegetarian proteins, fruits, vegetables, and whole grains.

- **don't be afraid to experiment**: Get creative in the kitchen, substitute ingredients, and discover what excites your taste buds.

- **Seek support**: Connect with other individuals following a similar path, share experiences, and draw strength from their journeys.

- **Celebrate the journey**: This is not a destination, it's a continuous exploration of delicious possibilities and empowered living.